The Fast Keto Diet

Dinner Recipe Book

Quick and Easy Tasty Recipes

Affordable for Busy People

Otis Fisher

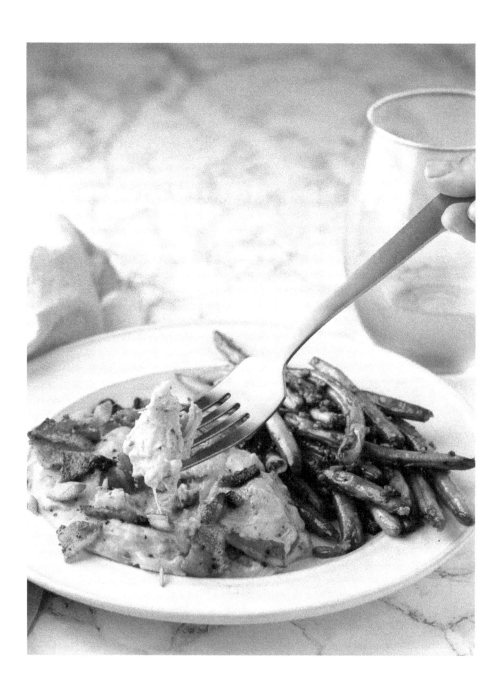

By reading this document, the reader agrees that under no circumstances is the author responsible for any losses, direct or indirect, which are incurred as a result of the use of information contained within this document, including, but not limited to, — errors, omissions, or inaccuracies.

Table of contents

Simple Blueberry Chaffle

Preparation Time: 7 minutes

Cooking Time: 3 minutes

Servings: 2

Ingredients:

- 1 Egg (beaten)
- 1/2 cup of Mozzarella cheese (grated)
- 1 tsp. Erythritol
- 1/2 tsp. Baking powder
- 1 tsp. Blueberry extract
- 1/2 tsp. Cinnamon
- 12 Blueberries (fresh)

Directions:

1. Heat the mini-Chaffle maker with Cooking spray before ready to use.
2. Mix the entire ingredient*s in a bowl (except the blueberries). You should also use a mixer to mix the ingredients.
3. Pour ample batter into the Chaffle maker's middle and fan it out to the corners. If you overfill the first one, fill it up a little less every time to prevent spilling. 6 new blueberries on top
4. Allow 3 1/2 minutes to Cooking with the lid closed.

5. Remove the chaffle and set it aside to cool for 5 minutes on a cooling rack; repeat for the second chaffle. Add a dollop of whipped cream and a couple new blueberries on top.

Nutrition:

Calories: 121

Carbohydrates: 3g

Protein: 9g

Fat: 8g

Cholesterol: 104mg

Sodium: 208mg

Sweet Keto Chaffles

Preparation Time: 7 minutes

Cooking Time: 10 minutes

Servings: 2

Ingredients:

- 1 large egg
- 1/2 cup of shredded low moisture mozzarella
- 1/4 cup of almond flour
- 1/8 tsp. of gluten-free baking powder
- 3 tbsp. of granulated low-carb sweetener such as Erythritol or Swerve or brown sugar substitute

Directions:

1. To make the Chaffles, measure out all of the ingredients. Using a standard Chaffle maker to preheat a mini Chaffle maker.
2. You may either mix all of the ingredients together in a bowl or blend them together. In a mixer or food processor, mix the egg, mozzarella, almond flour, and baking powder.
3. After that, stir in the sweetener. The dough would be a bit runnier if the sweetener is added before mixing, so I like to add mine after.
4. Spoon one-third of the batter (3 to 4 tsp., around 55 g/1.9 oz.) into the hot Chaffle maker to produce three tiny Chaffles.
5. Cooking for 3 to 4 minutes with the Chaffle maker closed.

6. When you're done, remove the lid and set it aside to cool for a few moments. Transfer the chaffle to a cooling rack softly with a spatula. Continue for the remaining hitter.

7. Allow the chaffles to cool fully before serving. When they're hot, they'll be fluffy, but when they cool, they'll crisp up. Top with full-fat milk, coconut yogurt, whipped cream, bananas, and/or bacon syrup for a low-carb dessert. Serve with One-Minute Chocolate Milk, hot or cold!

8. Enjoy right away, or keep the chaffles in a sealed jar at room temperature for up to 3 days, or in the fridge for up to a week, without any toppings. The jar will hold them fluffy, but if you like them crispy, you can leave them out.

Nutrition:

Protein: 45

Fat: 47

Carbohydrates: 8

Easy Keto Sandwich Bowl

Preparation Time: 10 minutes

Cooking Time: 0 minutes

Servings: 1

Ingredients:

- 5 slices smoked deli ham
- 1 cup of chopped romaine hearts
- 3 slices provolone cheese
- 3 pickles
- 4 banana peppers
- 1/2 cucumber
- 1/3 orange bell pepper
- 3 cherry tomatoes

Dressing:

- 2 tbsp. olive oil
- 4 tsp. red wine vinegar
- 1/4 tsp. Italian seasoning

Directions:

1. Place the ham, cheese, and vegetables in a bowl and chop them up.
2. Mix together the olive oil, red wine vinegar, and Italian seasoning.
3. Toss the keto sandwich bowl with some dressing.

4. Have fun! (To allow the oil/vinegar mixture to infuse all of the other ingredients, let the keto sandwich bowl sit for a few minutes.)

Nutrition

Calories: 1037

Carbohydrates: 14g

Protein: 62g

Fat: 80g

Cholesterol: 162mg

Sodium: 4458mg

Potassium: 1393mg

Open-Faced Grilled Ham and Cheese Sandwich

Preparation Time: 10 minutes

Cooking Time: 15 minutes

Servings: 1

Ingredients:

- Olive oil
- 4 slices white toasted sandwich bread
- 1 tbsp. mustard
- 4 slices Applegate Naturals Slow cooked Ham
- 4 slices Applegate Organics American Cheese
- 2 thickly sliced tomatoes
- 1 thinly sliced red onion
- Salt and freshly ground black pepper
- Finely chopped chives, for garnish

Directions:

1. Heat the oven to 400F. Using olive oil, coat a small sheet pan.
2. Arrange the toast slices on the plate. Cover every slice of toast with 1 slice of ham, 1 slice of cheese, 2 slices of tomato, and a few slices of red onion, and spread the mustard on top.
3. Drizzle olive oil over every sandwich and season lightly with salt and pepper.

4. Bake for 10-12 minutes, or until the cheese is bubbling and melted. Serve immediately with chives as a garnish.

Nutrition:

Calories: 147

Net Carb: 2.2g

Fat: 13g

Saturated Fat: 10.7g

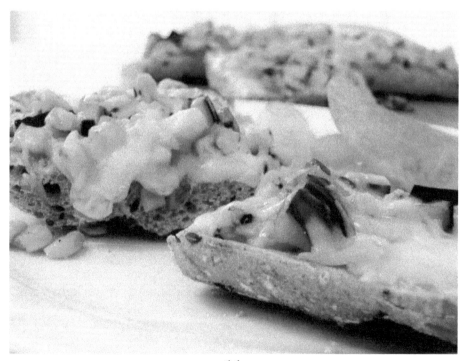

Cheesy Chaffle Sandwiches with Avocado and Bacon

Preparation Time: 10 minutes

Cooking Time: 25 minutes

Servings: 8

Ingredients:

- 10 large eggs
- 11/4 cups of shredded sharp Cheddar cheese
- 2 slices center-cut bacon, cooked and crumbled
- 1/2 tsp. ground pepper
- 2 small sliced avocados
- 2 small sliced tomatoes
- 4 large leaves butter head lettuce

Directions:

1. In a bowl, whisk the egg*s until creamy. Add the cheese, crumbled bacon, and pepper as need.
2. Cover a 7-inch round Chaffle iron (not Belgian) with Cooking spray and preheat it. 2/3 cup of the egg mixture should be poured onto the molten Chaffle iron. Cooking for 4 to 5 minutes, or until the eggs are set and light golden brown. Go on for the remainder of the egg mixture and Cooking oil in the same manner (making 4 chaffles total).
3. Every chaffle should be quartered. Half of the quarters can be covered in avocado slices, tomato slices, and lettuce

slices. Add the remaining chaffle quarters on to. Serve right away.

Nutrition:

Carbs 8 g

Fat 11 g

Protein 5 g

Calories 168

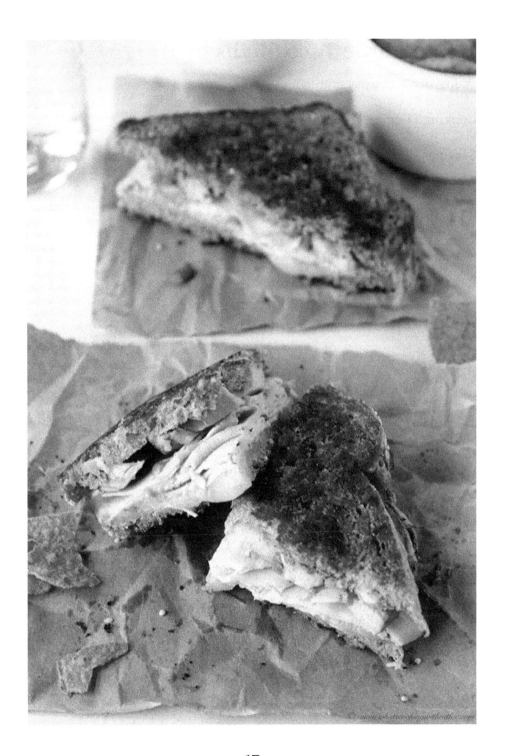

Keto Chaffle Taco Shells

Preparation Time: 5 minutes

Cooking Time: 20 minutes

Servings: 5

Ingredients:

- 1 tbsp. almond flour
- 1 cup of taco blend cheese
- 2 eggs
- 1/4 tsp. taco seasoning

Directions:

1. Mix almond flour, taco blend cheese, eggs, and taco seasoning in a mixing bowl. Using a fork, I find it easiest to mix anything.
2. At a point, pour 1.5 tsp. of taco chaffle batter into the Chaffle maker. In a Chaffle cooker, Cooking the chaffle batter for 4 minutes.
3. Remove the taco chaffle shell from the Chaffle maker and drape it over a bowl's rim. I used my pie pan because it was the only bowl I had on hand, but any bowl would suffice.
4. Continue to make chaffle taco shells before the batter runs out. Fill your taco shells with taco meat and your favorite toppings, and then dig in!

Nutrition:

Calories: 113

Carbohydrates: 1g

Protein: 8g

Fat: 9g

Cholesterol: 87mg

Sodium: 181mg

Taco Chaffle

Preparation Time: 5 minutes

Cooking Time: 10 minutes

Ingredients:

- 2 tbsp. coconut flour
- 1 tsp. baking powder
- 1/2 tsp. Himalayan pink salt
- 3 large eggs
- 1/2 cup of mozzarella cheese
- 1/2 cup of sharp cheddar cheese
- 1/2 Ib. ground beef
- 2 tsp. chili powder
- 1 tsp. cumin
- 1 tsp. paprika
- 1 tsp. garlic powder
- 1/4 cup of sour cream
- 1 diced ripe avocado
- 1/2 cup of diced tomato
- 1/2 cup of shredded romaine lettuce

Directions:

1. Merge flour, baking powder, and salt in a shallow mixing bowl.
2. Eggs should be beaten until frothy in a big mixing bowl.
3. Mix in the cheese until it is well mixed.
4. Mix with the dry ingredients.

5. Heat the Chaffle maker to medium high and liberally brush it with low carb Cooking oil.
6. Fill Chaffle maker halfway with batter, close, and Cooking for 4-5 minutes.
7. Brown the ground beef over medium-high pressure.
8. After the beef has been browned, add 14 cup of water and seasonings.
9. Stir well and Cooking for 7-9 minutes, or until water is absorbed, on low-medium heat.

Nutrition:

Cal: 216

Total: Fat: 20.9 g

Saturated Fat: 8.1 g

Cholesterol: 241 mg

Total Carbs: 8.3 g

Easy Double Chocolate Chaffles

Preparation Time: 1 minute

Cooking Time: 4 minutes

Servings: 1

Ingredients:

Double Chocolate Chaffles

- 1 eggs medium
- 1/2 cup of pre-shredded/grated mozzarella
- 1 tbsp. granulated sweetener of choice
- 1 tsp. vanilla
- 2 tbsp. almond meal/flour
- 1 tbsp. sugar-free chocolate chips/ cacao nibs
- 2 tbsp. cocoa powder unsweetened
- 1 tsp. heavy/double cream

Directions:

1. In a mixing bowl, mix the ingredients for your preferred flavor.
2. Preheat the Chaffle iron. Spray the mini-Chaffle maker with olive oil until it's warmed, and dump half the batter into it (or the entire batter into a large Chaffle maker).
3. Cooking for 2-4 minutes before removing and repeating the process. Per recipe, you should be able to make 2 mini-chaffles or 1 big chaffle.
4. Garnish, Cooking, and savor.

Nutrition:

Calories: 509

Carbohydrates: 5g

Fat: 45g

Protein: 23g

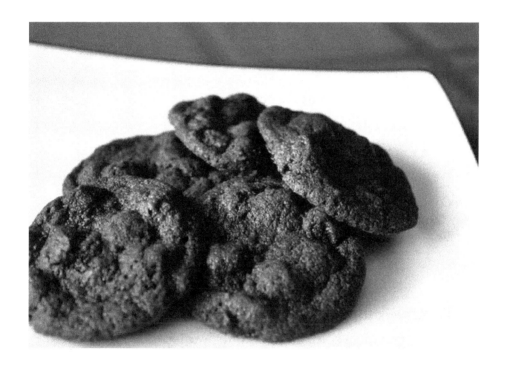

Pumpkin Chocolate Chip Chaffles

Preparation Time: 4 minutes

Cooking Time: 12 minutes

Servings: 3

Ingredients:

- 1/2 cup of shredded mozzarella cheese
- 4 tsp. pumpkin puree
- 1egg
- 2 tbsp. granulated swerve
- 1/4 tsp. pumpkin pie spice
- 4 tsp. sugar free chocolate chips
- 1 tbsp. almond flour

Directions:

1. Connect your Chaffle maker to the power source.
2. Mix the pumpkin puree and the egg in a small bowl. Make sure the pumpkin is thoroughly mixed with the egg.
3. Mix in the mozzarella cheese, almond flour, swerve, and pumpkin spice until thoroughly mixed.
4. After that, throw in your sugar-free chocolate chips.
5. Add part of the keto pumpkin pie to the mix. At a time, add chaffle mix to the Dish Mini Chaffle maker. In a Chaffle cooker, cook the chaffle batter for 4 minutes.
6. Cooking the second one after the first has finished Cooking.
7. Serve confectioners sweetener or whipped cream on top is a nice touch.

Nutrition:

Calories: 93

Carbohydrates: 2g

Protein: 7g

Fat: 7g

Cholesterol: 69mg

Sodium: 138mg

Potassium: 48mg

Fiber: 1g

Sugar: 1g

Keto Pizza Chaffle

Preparation Time: 4 minutes

Cooking Time: 6 minutes

Servings: 2

Ingredients:

- 1 egg
- 1/2 cup of mozzarella cheese
- 1 tbsp. pizza sauce
- 2 tbsp. sliced pepperoni
- 1/4 tsp. Italian seasoning

Directions:

1. Heat the Chaffle iron to medium-high.
2. Mix egg, mozzarella cheese, pizza sauce, pepperoni, and italian seasoning in a mixing bowl.
3. To make the pizza chaffle, mix all of the ingredients in a mixing bowl.
4. Pour the chaffle batter into the Chaffle irons middle. Close the Chaffle maker and then Cooking the Chaffle for 3-5 minutes, or until golden brown and set.
5. On the Chaffle iron, pizza chaffle ingredients are frying.
6. Remove the chaffle from the Chaffle maker and place it on a plate to eat.

Nutrition:

Calories: 141

Fat: 8.9g

Carbohydrates: 1.1g

Sugar: 0.2g

Protein: 13.5g

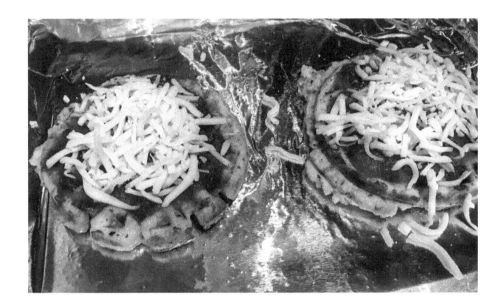

Mcgriddle Chaffle

Preparation Time: 3 minutes

Cooking Time: 7 minutes

Servings: 2

Ingredients:

- 3/4 cup of Shredded Mozzarella
- 1 Egg
- 1 tbsp. Sugar-Free Flavored Maple Syrup
- 1 tbsp. Monk fruit
- 1 Sausage Patty
- 1 Slice American Cheese

Directions:

1. Gather all of the necessary ingredients.
2. Heat the Dash Mini Chaffle Maker by plugging it in.
3. In a bowl, whisk together the egg.
4. Mix in the shredded Mozzarella, Swerve/Monk fruit, and Choc Zero Maple Syrup until smooth.
5. Place 2 tbsp. of the egg mixture in the Dash Mini Chaffle Maker, cover, and Cooking for 3–4 minutes. Rep before you've made as many Chaffles as you can.
6. Meanwhile, Cooking the sausage patty according to the package directions and melt the cheese on top while it's still warm.
7. Assemble Chaffle McGriddle and have a great time.

Nutrition:

Calories: 509

Carbohydrates: 5g

Fat: 45g

Protein: 23g

Jalapeno Chicken Popper Chaffle

Preparation Time: 3 minutes

Cooking Time: 25 minutes

Servings: 2

Ingredients:

- Canned chicken breast: 1/2 cup
- Onion powder: 1/8 tsp.
- Garlic powder: 1/8 tsp.
- Eggs: 1
- Cheddar cheese: 1/4 cup
- Jalapeno: 1 diced
- Cream cheese: 1 tbsp.
- Parmesan cheese: 1/8 tbsp.

Directions:

1. Preheat a mini Chaffle maker if needed and grease it
2. In a mixing bowl, beat eggs and add all the ingredients
3. Mix them all well
4. Pour the mixture to the lower plate of the Chaffle maker and spread it evenly to cover the plate properly
5. Close the lid
6. Cooking for at least 4 minutes to get the desired crunch
7. Remove the chaffle from the heat and keep aside for around one minute
8. Make as many chaffles as your mixture and Chaffle maker allow

9. Serve hot and enjoy!

Nutrition:

Cal: 216

Total: Fat: 20.9 g

Saturated Fat: 8.1 g

Cholesterol: 241 mg

Total Carbs: 8.3 g

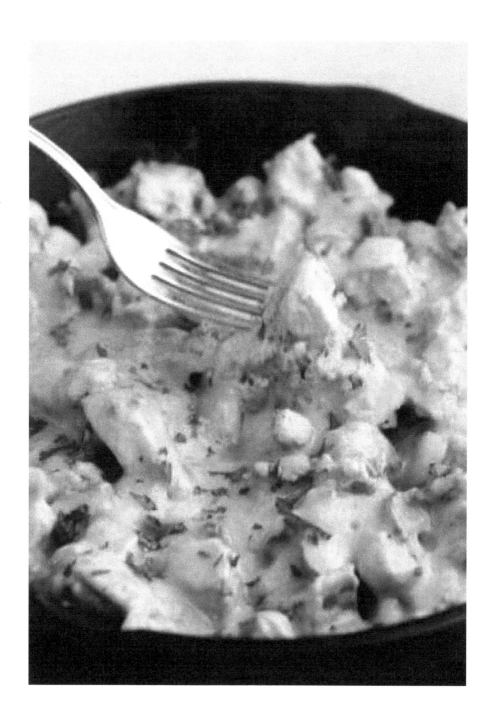

Cajun and Feta Chaffles

Preparation Time: 30 minutes

Cooking Time: 10 minutes

Servings: 1

Ingredients

- 1 egg white
- 1/4 cup shredded Mozzarella cheese
- 2 tbsps. almond flour
- 1 tsp. Cajun Seasoning

For Serving

- 1 egg
- 4 oz. feta cheese
- 1 tomato, sliced

Directions

1. Whisk together egg, cheese, and seasoning in a bowl.
2. Switch on and grease Chaffle maker with Cooking spray.
3. Pour batter in a preheated Chaffle maker.
4. Cooking chaffles for about 2-3 minutes until the chaffle is cooked through.
5. Meanwhile, fry the egg in a non-stick pan for about 1-2 minutes.
6. For serving set fried egg on chaffles with feta cheese and tomatoes slice.

Nutrition:

Calorie: 103

Protein: 7 g

Fat: 9 g

Carbohydrates: 1 g

Keto Tuna Melt Chaffle Recipe

Preparation time: 15 minutes

Cooking Time: 10 minutes

Serving: 2

Ingredients:

- Mozzarella cheese, one cup
- Eggs, two for adding into the chaffles
- Cheddar cheese, one cup
- Salt to taste
- Black pepper to taste
- Almond flour, 17 grams
- Shredded tuna, one cup
- Garlic powder, 17 grams
- Chopped cilantro, 17 grams

Directions:

1. Heat your Chaffle maker.
2. Always remember you heat your Chaffle maker till the point that it starts producing steam.
3. Remove the egg whites in a bowl and beat them to the point that they become fluffy.
4. Beat the egg yolks in a separate bowl.
5. Add in the egg yolks in the egg whites and delicately mix them with a spatula.
6. Combine the eggs and the rest of the ingredients except the chicken, cilantro and tzatziki sauce.

7. Add in the shredded chicken once the rest of the ingredients are well mixed.
8. When your Chaffle maker is heated adequately, pour in the mixture.
9. Close your Chaffle maker.
10. Let your chaffle Cooking for five to six minutes approximately.
11. When your chaffles are done, dish them out.
12. Add the chopped cilantro on top of the chaffles.
13. Your dish is ready to be served.

Nutrition:

Calories: 258

Fat: 19 g

Carbs: 5 g

Protein: 8 g

Fiber: 8 g

Cream Cheese Cookies

Preparation Time: 10 minutes

Cooking Time: 15 minutes

Servings: 10

Ingredients

- 1 egg white
- 1/4 cup butter, soft
- 3 cups almond flour
- 2 oz. cream cheese
- 2 tsp. vanilla extract
- 1/2 cup Erythritol

Directions

1. Beat together the butter, cream cheese, and Erythritol.
2. Add vanilla and egg white.
3. Gradually sift flour, 1/2 cup at a time into the mixture.
4. Set a baking sheet with parchment paper and spoon the cookies onto it.
5. Bake at 350F for 15 minutes.
6. Serve.

Nutrition:

Calories: 106

Fat: 9g

Carb: 3g

Protein: 3g

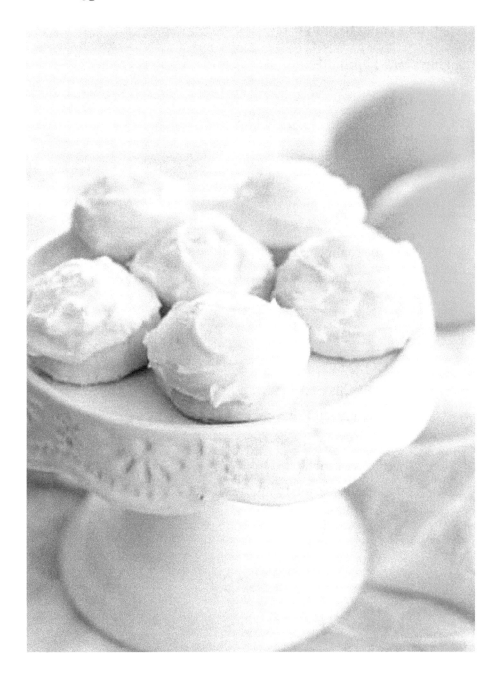

Chicken Mozzarella Chaffle

Preparation Time: 5 minutes

Cooking Time: 10 minutes

Servings: 2

Ingredients

- Chicken: 1 cup
- Egg: 2
- Mozzarella cheese: 1 cup and 4 tbsp.
- Tomato sauce: 6 tbsp.
- Basil: 1/2 tsp.
- Garlic: 1/2 tbsp.
- Butter: 1 tsp.

Directions:

1. In a pan, add butter and include small pieces of chicken to it
2. Stir for two minutes and then add garlic and basil
3. Set aside the cooked chicken
4. Preheat the mini Chaffle maker if needed
5. Mix cooked chicken, eggs, and 1 cup mozzarella cheese properly
6. Spread it to the mini Chaffle maker thoroughly
7. Cooking for 4 minutes or till it turns crispy and then remove it from the Chaffle maker
8. Make as many mini chaffles as you can

9. Now in a baking tray, line these mini chaffles and top with the tomato sauce and grated mozzarella cheese
10. Put the tray in the oven at 400 degrees until the cheese melts
11. Serve hot

Nutrition:

Cal: 216

Total: Fat: 20.9 g

Saturated Fat: 8.1 g

Cholesterol: 241 mg

Total Carbs: 8.3 g

Chicken Jamaican Jerk Chicken Chaffle

Preparation Time: 5 minutes

Cooking Time: 25 minutes

Servings: 2

Ingredients

For Chaffle:

- Egg: 2
- Mozzarella Cheese: 1 cup (shredded)
- Butter: 1 tbsp.
- Almond flour: 2 tbsp.
- Turmeric: 1/4 tsp.
- Baking powder: 1/4 tsp.
- Xanthan gum: a pinch
- Onion powder: a pinch
- Garlic powder: a pinch
- Salt: a pinch

For Chicken Jamaican Jerk:

- Organic ground chicken: 1 pound
- Dried thyme: 1 tsp.
- Garlic: 1 tsp. (granulated)
- Butter: 2 tbsp.
- Dried parsley: 2 tsp.
- Black pepper: 1/8 tsp.
- Salt: 1 tsp.

- Chicken broth: 1/2 cup
- Jerk seasoning: 2 tbsp.
- Onion: 1/2 medium chopped

Directions:

1. In a pan, melt butter and sauté onion
2. Add all the remaining ingredients of chicken Jamaican jerk and sauté
3. Now add chicken and chicken broth and stir
4. Cooking on medium-low heat for 10 minutes
5. Then Cooking on high heat and dry all the liquid
6. For chaffles, preheat a mini Chaffle maker if needed and grease it
7. In a mixing bowl, beat all the chaffle ingredients
8. Pour the mixture to the lower plate of the Chaffle maker and spread it evenly to cover the plate properly and close the lid
9. Cooking for at least 4 minutes to get the desired crunch
10. Remove the chaffle from the heat and keep aside for around one minute
11. Make as many chaffles as your mixture and Chaffle maker allow
12. Add the chicken in between of a chaffle and fold and enjoy

Nutrition:

Calories: 231

Carbohydrate: 2g

Fat: 18g

Protein: 13g

Chinese Five Spice Chicken Chaffles

Preparation Time: 5 minutes

Cooking Time: 15 minutes

Servings: 2

Ingredients

- Egg: 1
- Mozzarella cheese: 1/2 cup shredded
- Chinese five-spice: 1/2 tsp.
- Chicken: 1 cup boiled and shredded
- Garlic: 1 clove minced
- Onion powder: 1 tbsp.
- Salt: 1/2 tsp.

Directions:

1. Attach all the ingredients together and whisk well
2. Preheat your mini Chaffle iron if needed and grease it
3. Cooking your mixture in the mini Chaffle iron for at least 4 minutes
4. Make as many chaffles as you can

Nutrition:

Cal: 216

Total: Fat: 20.9 g

Saturated Fat: 8.1 g

Cholesterol: 241 mg

Total Carbs: 8.3 g

Fried Chicken Parmesan Chaffle

Preparation Time: 5 minutes

Cooking Time: 20 minutes

Servings: 2

Ingredients

- Cheddar cheese: 1/3 cup
- Egg: 1
- Baking powder: 1/4 teaspoon
- Flaxseed: 1 tsp. (ground)
- Parmesan cheese: 1/3 cup
- Chicken: 2 cm pieces cut boneless 1 cup
- Butter: 1 tbsp.
- Salt: as per your taste
- Black pepper: as per your taste

Directions:

1. Take a pan and heat butter
2. Add chicken and sprinkle salt and pepper and fry till soften
3. Mix cheddar cheese, egg, baking powder, and flaxseed in a bowl
4. Grease your Chaffle iron lightly
5. In your mini Chaffle iron, shred half of the parmesan cheese
6. Add a small amount of chaffle mixture to your mini Chaffle iron
7. Now add a layer of chicken
8. Again shred the remaining parmesan cheese on top

9. Cooking till the desired crisp is achieved
10. Make as many chaffles as your mixture and Chaffle maker allow

Nutrition:

Calories: 231

Carbohydrate: 2g

Fat: 18g

Protein: 13g

Chicken Green Chaffles

Preparation Time: 5 minutes

Cooking Time: 25 minutes

Servings: 4

Ingredients

- Chicken: 1/3 cup boiled and shredded
- Cabbage: 1/3 cup
- Broccoli: 1/3 cup
- Zucchini: 1/3 cup
- Egg: 2
- Mozzarella Cheese: 1 cup (shredded)
- Butter: 1 tbsp.
- Almond flour: 2 tbsp.
- Baking powder: 1/4 tsp.
- Onion powder: a pinch
- Garlic powder: a pinch
- Salt: a pinch

Directions:

1. In a deep saucepan, boil cabbage, broccoli, and zucchini for five minutes or till they tender, then strain, and blend
2. Mix all the remaining ingredients well together
3. Set a thin layer of the mixture on a preheated Chaffle iron
4. Add a layer of the blended vegetables on the mixture
5. Again add more mixture over the top
6. Cooking the chaffle for around 5 minutes

7. Serve with your favorite sauce

Nutrition:

Cal: 90

Carbs: 4g

Net Carbs: 2.5 g

Fiber: 4.5 g

Fat: 8 g

Buffalo Creamy Chicken Chaffle

Preparation Time: 5 minutes

Cooking Time: 10 minutes

Servings: 2

Ingredients

- Egg: 2
- Cheddar Cheese: 1 cup
- Buffalo sauce: 4 tbsp. or as per your taste
- Softened cream cheese: 1/4 cup
- Chicken: 1 cup
- Butter: 1 tsp.

Directions:

1. Heat the butter in the pan and add shredded chicken to it
2. Now remove from heat and add buffalo sauce as per your taste
3. In a bowl, add cooked chicken, cheddar cheese, softened cream cheese, and eggs
4. Mix all the ingredients well
5. Preheat the Chaffle maker and grease it
6. Now sprinkle a little cheddar cheese at the lower plate of the Chaffle maker
7. Spread your prepared batter evenly on the Chaffle maker
8. Now add a bit of cheese on the top as well and close the lid
9. Heat the chaffle for over 4 minutes or until it turns crispy

10. Make as many chaffles as your mixture and Chaffle maker allow

11. Serve hot with extra buffalo sauce

Nutrition:

Calories: 231

Carbohydrate: 2g

Fat: 18g

Protein: 13g

Artichoke and Spinach Chicken Chaffle

Preparation Time: 5 minutes

Cooking Time: 25 minutes

Servings: 2

Ingredients

- Chicken: 1/3 cup cooked and diced
- Spinach: 1/2 cup cooked and chopped
- Artichokes: 1/3 cup chopped
- Egg: 1
- Mozzarella Cheese: 1/3 cup (shredded)
- Cream cheese: 1 ounce
- Garlic powder: 1/4 tsp.

Directions:

1. Preheat a mini Chaffle maker if needed and grease it
2. In a mixing bowl, attach all the ingredients
3. Mix them all well
4. Pour the mixture to the lower plate of the Chaffle maker and spread it evenly to cover the plate properly
5. Close the lid
6. Cooking for at least 4 minutes to get the desired crunch
7. Remove the chaffle from the heat and keep aside for around one minute
8. Make as many chaffles as your mixture and Chaffle maker allow
9. Serve hot and enjoy!

Nutrition:

Calories 299

Fat 16g

Protein 23.4g

Carbs: 2

Garlic Chicken Chaffle

Preparation Time: 5 minutes

Cooking Time: 25 minutes

Servings: 2

Ingredients

- Chicken: 3-4 pieces
- Lemon juice: 1/2 tbsp.
- Garlic: 1 clove
- Kewpie mayo: 2 tbsp.
- Egg: 1
- Mozzarella cheese: 1/2 cup
- Salt: As per your taste

Directions:

1. In a pot, Cooking the chicken by adding one cup of water to it with salt and bring to boil
2. Close the lid of the pot and Cooking for 15-20 minutes
3. When done, remove from stove and shred the chicken pieces leaving the bones behind; discard the bones
4. Grate garlic finely into pieces
5. Beat the egg in the mixing bowl, add garlic, lemon juice, Kewpie mayo, and 1/8 cup of cheese
6. Preheat the Chaffle maker if needed and grease it
7. Attach the mixture to the Chaffle maker and Cooking for 4-5 minutes or until it is done
8. Remove the chaffles from the pan and preheat the oven

9. In the meanwhile, set the chaffles on a baking tray and spread the chicken on them
10. After that, sprinkle the remaining cheese on the chaffles
11. Set the tray in the oven and heat till the cheese melts
12. Serve hot
13. Make as many chaffles as you like

Nutrition:

Calories 465 Kcal

Total Fat 22.7g

Cholesterol 250.1mg

Sodium 1863.2mg

Total Carbohydrate 3.3g

Chicken Cauli Chaffle

Preparation Time: 5 minutes

Cooking Time: 25 minutes

Servings: 2

Ingredients

- Chicken: 3-4 pieces or 1/2 cup when done
- Soy Sauce: 1 tbsp.
- Garlic: 2 clove
- Cauliflower Rice: 1 cup
- Egg: 2
- Mozzarella cheese: 1 cup
- Salt: As per your taste
- Black pepper: 1/4 tsp.
- White pepper: 1/4 tsp. or as per your taste
- Green onion: 1 stalk

Directions:

1. Melt butter in oven or stove and set aside
2. In a pot, Cooking the chicken by adding one cup of water to it with salt and bring to boil
3. Close the lid of the pot and Cooking for 15-20 minutes
4. When done, remove from stove and shred the chicken pieces leaving the bones behind; discard the bones
5. Grate garlic finely into pieces
6. In a small bowl, whisk egg and mix chicken, garlic, cauliflower rice, soy sauce, black pepper, and white pepper

7. Mix all the ingredients well
8. Preheat the Chaffle maker if needed and grease it
9. Place around 1/8 cup of shredded mozzarella cheese to the Chaffle maker
10. Pour the mixture over the cheese on the Chaffle maker and add 1/8 cup shredded cheese on top as well
11. Cooking for 4-5 minutes or until it is done
12. Repeat and make as many chaffles as the batter can
13. Sprinkle chopped green onion on top and serve hot!

Nutrition:

Calories: 140

Fats: 12.7 g

Protein: 5.5 g

Net Carb: 0.1 g

Fiber: 0.2 g

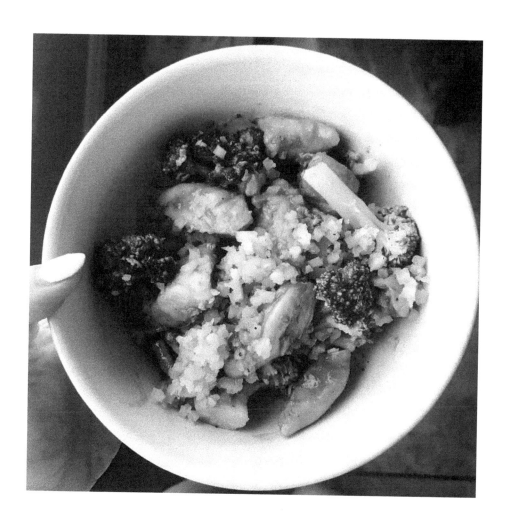

Easy Chicken Halloumi Burger Chaffle

Preparation Time: 5 minutes

Cooking Time: 25 minutes

Servings: 2

Ingredients

For the Chaffle:

- Egg: 2
- Mozzarella Cheese: 1 cup (shredded)
- Butter: 1 tbsp.
- Almond flour: 2 tbsp.
- Baking powder: 1/4 tsp.
- Onion powder: a pinch
- Garlic powder: a pinch
- Salt: a pinch

For the Chicken Patty:

- Ground chicken: 1 lb.
- Onion powder: 1/2 tbsp.
- Garlic powder: 1/2 tbsp.
- Halloumi cheese: 1 cup
- Salt: 1/4 tsp. or as per your taste
- Black pepper: 1/4 tsp.

For Serving:

- Lettuce leaves: 2
- American cheese: 2 slices

Directions:

1. Mix the entire chicken patty ingredient in a bowl
2. Make equal-sized patties; either grill them or fry them
3. Preheat a mini Chaffle maker if needed and grease it
4. In a mixing bowl, add all the chaffle ingredients and mix well
5. Pour the mixture to the lower plate of the Chaffle maker and spread it evenly to cover the plate properly and close the lid
6. Cooking for at least 4 minutes to get the desired crunch
7. Remove the chaffle from the heat and keep aside for around one minute
8. Make as many chaffles as your mixture and Chaffle maker allow
9. Serve with the chicken patties, lettuce, and a cheese slice in between of two chaffles

Nutrition

Calories: 1037

Carbohydrates: 14g

Protein: 62g

Fat: 80g

Cholesterol: 162mg

Simple Chicken Cheese Chaffle

Preparation time: 5 minutes

Cooking Time: 10 minutes

Serving: 2

Ingredients:

- Chicken: 1 cup
- Egg: 2
- Mozzarella cheese: 1 cup and 4 tbsp.
- Tomato sauce: 6 tbsp.
- Basil: 1/2 tsp.
- Garlic: 1/2 tbsp.
- Butter: 1 tsp.

Directions:

1. In a pan, add butter and include small pieces of chicken to it
2. Stir for two minutes and then add garlic and basil
3. Set aside the cooked chicken
4. Preheat the mini Chaffle maker if needed
5. Mix cooked chicken, eggs, and 1 cup mozzarella cheese properly
6. Spread it to the mini Chaffle maker thoroughly
7. Cooking for 4 minutes or till it turns crispy and then remove it from the Chaffle maker

8. Make as many mini chaffles as you can
9. Now in a baking tray, line these mini chaffles and top with the tomato sauce and grated mozzarella cheese
10. Put the tray in the oven at 400 degrees until the cheese melts
11. Serve hot

Nutrition:

Carbs 8 g

Fat 11 g

Protein 5 g

Calories 168

Jamaican Jerk Chicken Chaffle

Preparation time: 5 minutes

Cooking Time: 15 minutes

Serving: 2

Ingredients:

For Chaffle:

- Egg: 2
- Mozzarella Cheese: 1 cup (shredded)
- Butter: 1 tbsp.
- Almond flour: 2 tbsp.
- Turmeric: 1/4 tsp.
- Baking powder: 1/4 tsp.
- Xanthan gum: a pinch
- Onion powder: a pinch
- Garlic powder: a pinch
- Salt: a pinch

For Chicken Jamaican Jerk:

- Organic ground chicken: 1 pound
- Dried thyme: 1 tsp.
- Garlic: 1 tsp. (granulated)
- Butter: 2 tbsp.
- Dried parsley: 2 tsp.
- Black pepper: 1/8 tsp.
- Salt: 1 tsp.

- Chicken broth: 1/2 cup
- Jerk seasoning: 2 tbsp.
- Onion: 1/2 medium chopped

Directions:

1. In a pan, melt butter and sauté onion
2. Add all the remaining ingredients of chicken Jamaican jerk and sauté
3. Now add chicken and chicken broth and stir
4. Cooking on medium-low heat for 10 minutes
5. Then Cooking on high heat and dry all the liquid
6. For chaffles, preheat a mini Chaffle maker if needed and grease it
7. In a mixing bowl, beat all the chaffle ingredients
8. Pour the mixture to the lower plate of the Chaffle maker and spread it evenly to cover the plate properly and close the lid
9. Cooking for at least 4 minutes to get the desired crunch
10. Remove the chaffle from the heat and keep aside for around one minute
11. Make as many chaffles as your mixture and Chaffle maker allow
12. Add the chicken in between of a chaffle and fold and enjoy

Nutrition:

Calories 292

Fat 26g

Protein 13.4g

Carbs: 3.4

Healthy Chicken Chaffles

Preparation time: 5 minutes

Cooking Time: 10 minutes

Serving: 4

Ingredients:

For Chaffle:

- Chicken: 1/3 cup boiled and shredded
- Cabbage: 1/3 cup
- Broccoli: 1/3 cup
- Zucchini: 1/3 cup
- Egg: 2
- Mozzarella Cheese: 1 cup (shredded)
- Butter: 1 tbsp.
- Almond flour: 2 tbsp.
- Baking powder: 1/4 tsp.
- Onion powder: a pinch
- Garlic powder: a pinch
- Salt: a pinch

Directions

1. In a deep saucepan, boil cabbage, broccoli, and zucchini for five minutes or till it tenders, strain, and blend
2. Mix all the remaining ingredients well together
3. Pour a thin layer on a preheated Chaffle iron
4. Add a layer of the blended vegetables on the mixture
5. Again add more mixture over the top

6. Cooking the chaffle for around 5 minutes
7. Serve with your favorite sauce

Nutrition:

Calories: 231

Carbohydrate: 2g

Fat: 18g

Protein: 13g

Buffalo Chicken Chaffle

Preparation time: 5 minutes

Cooking Time: 10 minutes

Serving: 2

Ingredients:

- Egg: 2
- Cheddar Cheese: 1 cup
- Buffalo sauce: 4 tbsp. or as per your taste
- Softened cream cheese: 1/4 cup
- Chicken: 1 cup
- Butter: 1 tsp.

Directions:

1. Heat the butter in the pan and add shredded chicken to it
2. Now remove from heat and add buffalo sauce as per your taste
3. In a bowl, add cooked chicken, cheddar cheese, softened cream cheese, and eggs
4. Mix all the ingredients well
5. Preheat the Chaffle maker and grease it
6. Now sprinkle a little cheddar cheese at the lower plate of the Chaffle maker
7. Spread your prepared batter evenly on the Chaffle maker
8. Now add a bit of cheese on the top as well and close the lid
9. Heat the chaffle for over 4 minutes or until it turns crispy

10. Make as many chaffles as your mixture and Chaffle maker allow

11. Serve hot with extra buffalo sauce

Nutrition:

Calories: 147

Net Carb: 2.2g

Fat: 13g

Saturated Fat: 10.7g

Garlic Spicy Chicken Chaffle

Preparation time: 15 minutes

Cooking Time: 10 minutes

Serving: 2

Ingredients:

- Chicken: 3-4 pieces
- Lemon juice: 1/2 tbsp.
- Garlic: 1 clove
- Kewpie mayo: 2 tbsp.
- Egg: 1
- Mozzarella cheese: 1/2 cup
- 1/2chili powder
- Salt: As per your taste

Directions:

1. In a pot, Cooking the chicken by adding one cup of water to it with salt and bring to boil
2. Close the lid of the pot and Cooking for 15-20 minutes
3. When done, remove from stove and shred the chicken pieces leaving the bones behind; discard the bones
4. Grate garlic finely into pieces
5. Beat the egg in the mixing bowl, add garlic, lemon juice, Kewpie mayo, and 1/8 cup of cheese
6. Preheat the Chaffle maker if needed and grease it
7. Attach the mixture to the Chaffle maker and Cooking for 4-5 minutes or until it is done

8. Remove the chaffles from the pan and preheat the oven

9. In the meanwhile, set the chaffles on a baking tray and spread the chicken on them

10. After that, sprinkle the remaining cheese on the chaffles

11. Set the tray in the oven and heat till the cheese melts

12. Serve hot

13. Make as many chaffles as you like

Nutrition:

Protein: 31

Fat: 66

Carbohydrates: 2

Easy Halloumi Burger Chaffle

Preparation time: 15 minutes

Cooking Time: 20 minutes

Serving: 2

Ingredients:

For the Chaffle:

- Egg: 2
- Mozzarella Cheese: 1 cup (shredded)
- Butter: 1 tbsp.
- Almond flour: 2 tbsp.
- Baking powder: 1/4 tsp.
- Onion powder: a pinch
- Garlic powder: a pinch
- Salt: a pinch

For the Chicken Patty:

- Ground chicken: 1 lb.
- Onion powder: 1/2 tbsp.
- Garlic powder: 1/2 tbsp.
- Halloumi cheese: 1 cup
- Salt: 1/4 tsp. or as per your taste
- Black pepper: 1/4 tsp.

For Serving:

- Lettuce leaves: 2
- American cheese: 2 slices

Directions:

1. Mix the entire chicken patty ingredient in a bowl
2. Make equal-sized patties; either grill them or fry them
3. Preheat a mini Chaffle maker if needed and grease it
4. In a mixing bowl, add all the chaffle ingredients and mix well
5. Pour the mixture to the lower plate of the Chaffle maker and spread it evenly to cover the plate properly and close the lid
6. Cooking for at least 4 minutes to get the desired crunch
7. Remove the chaffle from the heat and keep aside for around one minute
8. Make as many chaffles as your mixture and Chaffle maker allow.
9. Serve with the chicken patties, lettuce, and a cheese slice in between of two chaffles

Nutrition:

Carbs: 12 g

Fat: 1 g

Protein: 2 g

Calories: 57

Healthy Chicken Eggplant Chaffle

Preparation time: 15 minutes

Cooking Time: 10 minutes

Serving: 2

Ingredients:

For Chaffles:

- Eggs: 2
- Cheddar cheese: 1/2 cup
- Parmesan cheese: 2 tbsp.
- Italian season: 1/4 tsp.
- Chicken: 1 cup

For Eggplant:

- Eggplant: 1 big
- Salt: 1 pinch
- Black pepper: 1 pinch

Directions:

1. Boil the chicken in water for 15 minutes and strain
2. Shred the chicken into small pieces and set aside
3. Cut the eggplant in slices and boil in water and strain
4. Add a pinch of salt and pepper
5. Add all the chaffle ingredients in a bowl and mix well to make a mixture
6. Add the boiled chicken as well
7. Preheat a mini Chaffle maker if needed and grease it

8. Pour the mixture to the lower plate of the Chaffle maker and spread it evenly to cover the plate properly

9. Add the eggplant over two slices on the mixture and cover the lid

10. Cooking for at least 4 minutes to get the desired crunch

11. Remove the chaffle from the heat and keep aside for around one minute

12. Make as many chaffles as your mixture and Chaffle maker allow

13. Serve hot with your favorite sauce

Nutrition:

Calories 69 Kcal

Total Fat 5g

Cholesterol 67.4mg

Sodium 874.7mg

Total Carbohydrate 2.7g

Ginger Chicken Cucumber Chaffle Roll

Preparation time: 20 minutes

Cooking Time: 10 minutes

Serving: 2

Ingredients:

For Garlic Chicken:

- Chicken mince: 1 cup
- Salt: 1/4 tsp. or as per your taste
- Black pepper: 1/4 tsp.
- Lemon juice: 1 tbsp.
- Butter: 2 tbsp.
- Garlic juvenile: 2 tbsp.
- Garlic powder: 1 tsp.
- Soy sauce: 1 tbsp.

For Chaffle:

- Egg: 2
- Mozzarella cheese: 1 cup (shredded)
- Garlic powder: 1 tsp.
- For Serving:
- Cucumber: 1/2 cup (diced)
- Parsley: 1 tbsp.

Directions:

1. In a frying pan, melt butter and add juvenile garlic and sauté for 1 minute

2. Now add chicken mince and Cooking till it tenders
3. When done, add rest of the ingredients and set aside
4. In a mixing bowl, beat eggs and add mozzarella cheese to them with garlic powder
5. Mix them all well and pour to the greasy mini Chaffle maker
6. Cooking for at least 4 minutes to get the desired crunch
7. Remove the chaffle from the heat, add the chicken mixture in between with cucumber and fold
8. Make as many chaffles as your mixture and Chaffle maker allow
9. Serve hot and top with parsley

Nutrition:

Calories 90 Kcal

Fats 3.32g

Carbs 2.97g

Net carbs 2.17g

Protein 12.09g

Carbquik Chaffles

Preparation time: 20 minutes

Cooking Time: 20 minutes

Serving: 20

Ingredients:

- 1/2 cup egg substitute
- 1-3/4 cups almond milk
- 1/2 cup fat-free plain yogurt
- 1 tablespoon vanilla extract
- 2 cup Carbquik
- 1/2 cup sugar
- 2 tablespoons sugar
- 1/2 cup mozzarella cheese, shredded
- 4 teaspoons baking powder
- 1/4 teaspoon salt

Directions:

1. In a large bowl, set egg substitute until frothy.
2. Merge in the milk, yogurt and vanilla.
3. Add mozzarella cheese and stir well.
4. Combine Carbquik, sugar substitute, baking powder and salt
5. Stir into almond milk mixture just until blend.
6. Set in a preheated Chaffle iron according to manufacturer's directions until golden brown.

Nutrition:

Calories 132,

Total Fat 18 g,

Cholesterol 2 mg,

Sodium 273 mg,

Total Carbohydrate 9 g,

Protein 16 g,

Fiber 2 g

Chicken Jalapeno Chaffle

Preparation time: 20 minutes

Cooking Time: 15 minutes

Serving: 2

Ingredients:

- Egg: 2
- Cheddar cheese: 11/2 cup
- Deli Jalapeno: 16 slices
- Boiled chicken: 1 cup (shredded)

Directions:

1. Preheat a mini Chaffle maker if needed
2. In a mixing bowl, beat eggs and add chicken and half cheddar cheese to them
3. Mix them all well
4. Shred some of the remaining cheddar cheese to the lower plate of the Chaffle maker
5. Now pour the mixture to the shredded cheese
6. Add the cheese again on the top with around 4 slices of jalapeno and close the lid
7. Cooking for at least 4 minutes to get the desired crunch
8. Serve hot
9. Make as many chaffles as your mixture allows

Nutrition:

Calories: 153

Fat: 12.2g

Carbohydrates: 0.7g

Sugar: 0.4g

Protein: 10.3g

Chicken Stuffed Chaffles

Preparation time: 20 minutes

Cooking Time: 20 minutes

Serving: 2

Ingredients:

For Chaffle:

- Egg: 2
- Mozzarella Cheese: 1/2 cup (shredded)
- Garlic powder: 1/4 tsp.
- Salt: 1/4 tsp. or as per your taste
- Black pepper: 1/4 tsp.

For Stuffing:

- Onion: 1 small diced
- Chicken: 1 cup
- Butter: 4 tbsp.
- Salt: 1/4 tsp. or as per your taste
- Black pepper: 1/4 tsp.

Directions:

1. Preheat a mini Chaffle maker if needed and grease it
2. In a mixing bowl, add all the chaffle ingredients
3. Mix them all well
4. Pour the mixture to the lower plate of the Chaffle maker and spread it evenly to cover the plate properly and close the lid
5. Cooking for at least 4 minutes to get the desired crunch

6. Remove the chaffle from the heat and keep aside
7. Make as many chaffles as your mixture and Chaffle maker allow
8. Take a small frying pan and melt butter in it on medium-low heat
9. Sauté chicken and onion and add salt and pepper
10. Take another bowl and tear chaffles down into minute pieces
11. Add chicken and onion to it
12. Take a casserole dish, and add this new stuffing mixture to it
13. Bake it at 350 degrees for around 30 minutes and serve hot

Nutrition:

Calories: 141

Fat: 8.9g

Carbohydrates: 1.1g

Sugar: 0.2g

Protein: 13.5g

Easy Chicken Vegetable Chaffles

Preparation time: 20 minutes

Cooking Time: 10 minutes

Serving: 2

Ingredients:

For the Chaffle:

- Egg: 2
- Mozzarella Cheese: 1 cup (shredded)
- Salt: a pinch

For the Chicken:

- Chicken pieces: 2-4
- Ginger powder: 1/2 tbsp.
- Salt: 1/4 tsp. or as per your taste
- Black pepper: 1/4 tsp.
- Cauliflower: 3 tbsp.
- Cabbage: 3 tbsp.
- Green pepper: 1 tbsp.
- Spring onion: 1 stalk

Directions:

1. Boil the chicken, green pepper, cauliflower, and cabbage in saucepan, when done strain the water
2. Shred the chicken into small pieces and blend all the vegetables and mix them together

3. Finely divide the spring onion and mix with the chicken and set aside
4. Preheat a mini Chaffle maker if needed and grease it
5. In a mixing bowl, add all the chaffle ingredients and mix well
6. Pour a little amount of mixture to the lower plate of the Chaffle maker and spread it evenly to cover the plate properly
7. Add the chicken mixture on top and again spread the thin layer of mixture and close the lid
8. Cooking for at least 4 minutes to get the desired crunch
9. Remove the chaffle from the heat
10. Make as many chaffles as your mixture and Chaffle maker allow
11. Serve hot and enjoy

Nutrition:

Cal: 90

Carbs: 4g

Net Carbs: 2.5 g

Fiber: 4.5 g

Fat: 8 g

Protein: 8g

Sugars: 3 g

Cabbage Chicken Chaffle:

Preparation time: 5 minutes

Cooking Time: 10 minutes

Serving: 2

Ingredients:

- Chicken: 3-4 pieces or 1/2 cup when done
- Soy Sauce: 1 tbsp.
- Garlic: 2 clove
- Cabbage: 1 cup
- Egg: 2
- Mozzarella cheese: 1 cup
- Salt: As per your taste
- Black pepper: 1/4 tsp.
- White pepper: 1/4 tsp. or as per your taste

Directions:

1. Melt butter in oven or stove and set aside
2. In a pot, Cooking the chicken and cabbage by adding one cup of water to it with salt and bring to boil
3. Close the lid of the pot and Cooking for 15-20 minutes
4. When done, remove from stove and shred the chicken pieces leaving the bones behind; discard the bones
5. Strain water from cabbage and blend
6. Grate garlic finely into pieces
7. In a small bowl, set egg and mix chicken, cabbage, garlic, soy sauce, black pepper, and white pepper

8. Mix all the ingredients well
9. Preheat the Chaffle maker if needed and grease it
10. Place around 1/8 cup of shredded mozzarella cheese to the Chaffle maker
11. Pour the mixture over the cheese on the Chaffle maker and add 1/8 cup shredded cheese on top as well
12. Cooking for 4-5 minutes or until it is done
13. Make as many chaffles as your mixture and Chaffle maker allow
14. Serve hot!

Nutrition:

Calories: 266

Carbohydrates: 2g

Fat: 23g

Protein: 13g

Chicken Spinach Chaffle

Preparation time: 15 minutes

Cooking Time: 30 minutes

Serving: 2

Ingredients:

- Spinach: 1/2 cup
- Chicken: 1/2 cup boneless
- Egg: 1
- Shredded mozzarella: half cup
- Pepper: As per your taste
- Garlic powder: 1 tbsp.
- Onion powder: 1 tbsp.
- Salt: As per your taste
- Basil: 1 tsp.

Directions:

1. Boil chicken in water to make it tender
2. Shred-it into small pieces and set aside
3. Boil spinach in a saucepan for 10 minutes and strain
4. Preheat your Chaffle iron
5. Add all the ingredients to boiled spinach in a bowl and mix well
6. Now add the shredded chicken
7. Grease your Chaffle iron lightly
8. Pour the mixture into a full-size Chaffle maker and spread evenly

9. Cooking till it turns crispy
10. Make as many chaffles as your mixture and Chaffle maker allow
11. Serve crispy and with your favorite keto sauce

Nutrition:

Calories 465 Kcal

Total Fat 22.7g

Cholesterol 250.1mg

Sodium 1863.2mg

Total Carbohydrate 3.3g

Chicken BBQ Chaffle

Preparation time: 15 minutes

Cooking Time: 15 minutes

Serving: 2

Ingredients:

- Chicken: 1/2 cup
- Butter: 1 tbsp.
- BBQ sauce: 1 tbsp. (sugar-free)
- Almond flour: 2 tbsp.
- Egg: 1
- Cheddar cheese: 1/2 cup

Directions:

1. Cooking the chicken in the butter on a low-medium heat for 10 minutes
2. Preheat your Chaffle iron
3. In mixing bowl, add all the chaffle ingredients including chicken and mix well
4. Grease your Chaffle iron lightly
5. Pour the mixture to the bottom plate evenly; also spread it out to get better results and close the upper plate and heat
6. Cooking for 6 minutes or until the chaffle is done
7. Make as many chaffles as your mixture and Chaffle maker allow

Nutrition:

Calories: 231

Carbohydrate: 2g

Fat: 18g

Protein: 13g

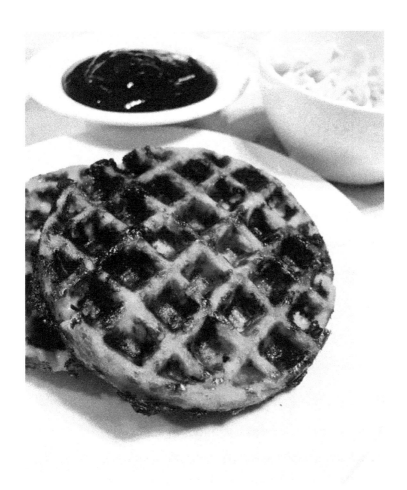

Crispy Fried Chicken Chaffle

Preparation time: 15 minutes

Cooking Time: 25 minutes

Serving: 2

Ingredients:

For Chaffle:

- Egg: 1
- Mozzarella Cheese: 1/2 cup (shredded)

For Fried Chicken:

- Chicken strips: 8 pieces
- Butter: 2 tbsp.
- Salt: 1/4 tsp. or as per your taste
- Black pepper: 1/4 tsp.
- Red chili flakes: 1/2 tsp.

Directions:

1. In a frying pan, dissolve butter and fry chicken strips on medium-low heat
2. Add the spices at the end and set aside
3. Mix all the chaffle ingredients well together
4. Pour a thin layer on a preheated Chaffle iron
5. Add chicken strips and pour again more mixture over the top
6. Cooking the chaffle for around 5 minutes

7. Make as many chaffles as your mixture and Chaffle maker allow
8. Serve hot!

Nutrition:

Calories 316 Kcal

Fats 21.78g

Carbs 6.52g

Everything Chaffle

Preparation time: 8 minutes

Cooking time: 10 minutes

Servings: 2

Ingredients:

- 1 Large Egg
- 1 Ounce 6 Cheese Italian Blend Cheese, Finely Shredded
- 3 Tablespoons Almond Flour
- 1 Pinch Salt
- Butter Flavored Non-Stick Cooking Spray
- Topping
- 2 Ounces Cream Cheese
- 2 Teaspoons Everything Bagel Seasoning

Directions:

1. Plugin the mini Chaffle maker and preheat it. There is a light for many Chaffle makers to indicate when it is preheated. Be sure that it is completely heated before continuing for the best results.
2. Crack the large egg into a small bowl and beat vigorously with a fork until well-mixed yolk and white.
3. Chop the shredded Italian cheese into smaller pieces using a small chopping board and medium-sized knife. It ensures that the cheese can be distributed more evenly throughout the egg mixture.

4. Add the egg mixture with the butter, almond flour and salt and whisk with a fork until all is well mixed.
5. Sprinkle Chaffle maker with non-stick Cooking spray flavored with butter.
6. Put 1/2 of the mixture in a miniature Chaffle maker's grill center. Stretch the mixture to the grill edges and close the Chaffle maker.
7. Cooking the chaffle for 5 minutes or brown and Cooking through until toasty.
8. Gently remove the chaffle using a small fork and place it to cool on a sheet of paper towels.
9. Spray Chaffle maker with non-stick Cooking spray flavored with butter and Cooking the remaining mixture of the chaffle the same as the first.
10. When they cool down, chaffles will become crisper.
11. Layer cream cheese chaffles and sprinkle with bagel seasoning.

Nutrition:

Calories: 249kcal

Carbohydrates: 5g

Protein: 11g

Fat: 22g

Saturated Fat: 7g

Cholesterol: 116mg

Cheesy Salmon Chaffles

Preparation time: 5 minutes

Cooking time: 7 minutes

Serving: 2

Ingredient

- 2 Basic Savory Chaffles
- 1/4 cup cream cheese
- 2 to 3 slices smoked salmon
- 1 tablespoon chopped chives
- Pinch of black pepper

Direction

1. Prepare a batch of the Basic Savory Chaffles by following the instructions of the first recipe.
2. Let the chaffles cool down and spread the cream cheese and smoked salmon on top. Sprinkle with the chives and black pepper.
3. Serve immediately.

Nutrition

Calories: 332

Fat: 28.1g

Protein: 19.7g

Wholesome Keto Chaffles

Preparation time: 5 minutes

Cooking time: 5 minutes

Serving: 12

Ingredient

- 1 cup almond flour
- 3 tablespoons ground flaxseed
- 3 teaspoons baking powder
- 1/2 teaspoon salt
- 2 eggs, separated
- 1/2 cup mozzarella cheese, shredded
- 2 cups almond milk
- 3 tablespoons canola oil
- 3 tablespoons unsweetened applesauce
- Mixed fresh berries, optional

Directions:

1. In a large bowl, merge the flour, flax, baking powder and salt.
2. Combine the egg yolks, almond milk, oil and applesauce.
3. Stir into dry ingredients until just moistened.
4. In a small bowl, merge egg whites until stiff peaks form; fold into batter.
5. Add mozzarella cheese and stir well.
6. Set in a preheated Chaffle iron until golden brown.
7. Set with berries if desired.

Nutrition:

Calories 278,

Total Fat 19 g,

Cholesterol 70 mg,

Sodium 456 mg,

Total Carbohydrate 11 g,

Protein 18 g, Fiber 4 g

Keto Cajun Shrimp and Avocado Chaffle Recipe

Preparation time: 25 minutes

Cooking Time: 20 minutes

Serving: 2

Ingredients:

- Mozzarella cheese, one cup
- Eggs, two for adding into the chaffles

For patties:

- Chopped fresh cilantro, 20 grams
- Egg, one
- Salt to taste
- Black pepper to taste
- Ground shrimp, half pound
- Cajun seasoning, 17 grams
- For garnish:
- Avocado slices, half cup
- Lettuce leaf, two

For the sauce:

- Soy sauce, 17 grams
- Japanese sake, 34 grams
- Xanthan gum, 5 grams

Directions:

1. Heat your Chaffle maker.

2. Always remember you heat your Chaffle maker till the point that it starts producing steam.
3. Remove the egg whites in a bowl and beat them to the point that they become fluffy.
4. Beat the egg yolks in a separate bowl.
5. Add in the egg yolks in the egg whites and delicately mix them with a spatula.
6. Combine the eggs and cheese.
7. When your Chaffle maker is heated adequately, pour in the mixture.
8. Close your Chaffle maker.
9. Let your chaffle Cooking for five to six minutes approximately.
10. When your chaffles are done, dish them out.
11. In the meanwhile, mix all the ingredients for the sauce in a bowl.
12. Mix the ingredients for the patties.
13. Make small two patties and fry them in olive oil until they are done.
14. Lay a lettuce leaf on the chaffle, add the patty and place the avocado slices on top.
15. Pour the sauce on top and close your sandwich.
16. Your dish is ready to be served.

Nutrition:

Cal: 203

Carbs: 5 g

Fats 2.7 g

Protein 5.2 g

Fiber: 1 g

Pumpkin Chaffle with Cream Cheese Frosting

Preparation Time: 3 minutes

Cooking Time: 8 minutes

Servings: 2

Ingredients:

- 1 egg
- 1/2 cup of mozzarella cheese
- 1/2 tsp. pumpkin pie spice
- 1 tbs. pumpkin solid packed with no sugar added
- Optional Cream Cheese Frosting Ingredients:
- 2 tbs. softened and room temperature cream cheese
- 2 tbs. any of your favorite keto-friendly sweetener
- 1/2 tsp. clear extract of vanilla

Directions:

1. Heat the mini Chaffle maker.
2. Whip the egg in a little bowl.
3. Mix the cheese, pumpkin pie spice, and pumpkin in a mixing bowl.
4. Mix well.
5. Cooking for at least 3 to 4 minutes, until golden brown, in the mini Chaffle maker with half of the mixture.
6. When the chaffle is baking, mix all of the ingredients for the cream cheese frosting in a mixing bowl and whisk until smooth and fluffy.

7. Serve the hot chaffle with the cream cheese frosting right away.

Nutrition:

Calories: 266

Carbohydrates: 2g

Fat: 23g

Protein: 13g

Chaffle Bread Pudding With Cranberries

Preparation Time: 10 minutes

Cooking Time: 30 minutes

Servings: 2

Ingredients:

Chaffles:

- 4 eggs
- 1 cup of shredded part skim mozzarella - cheese

Pudding:

- 3 beaten eggs
- 2 tsp. extract of vanilla
- 2 tsp. pumpkin pie spice
- 1/4 cup of So Nourished Erythritol sweetener blend
- 1/2 cup of canned pumpkin
- 1/2 cup of heavy cream
- 1/2 cup of fresh or frozen cranberries
- 1 tbsp. granulated Erythritol to sprinkle on top

Directions:

Chaffles:

1. Heat the Chaffle maker
2. In a mixing bowl, merge together the eggs and grated cheese.
3. Cooking chaffles in a Chaffle maker; depending on the unit, you'll get 4-6 chaffles/Chaffles.

4. Cooking 1/4 cup of batter at a time in a mini Chaffle machine (3-4 minutes every)
5. You can cook all of the batter at once in a full-size Chaffle maker for around 7 minutes.
6. Allow chaffles to cool on a rack before serving.

Bread Pudding:

1. Heat the oven to 350F. Tear the chaffles into bite-size bits with your hands.
2. Mix beaten eggs, milk, pumpkin, vanilla, spice blend, and sweetener in a mixing bowl.
3. To mix, whisk all together thoroughly.
4. Pour onto a pie plate that has been greased.
5. Top with cranberries and a little sugar if needed (if desired)
6. Heat oven to 350F and bake for 30 minutes, or until set.
7. Serve warm or cold with ice cream on top (if desired)

Nutrition:

Calories: 160

Total Fat: 12g

Cholesterol: 24mg

Sodium: 93mg

Carbohydrates: 4g

Fiber: 1g

Sugar: 1g

Protein: 9g

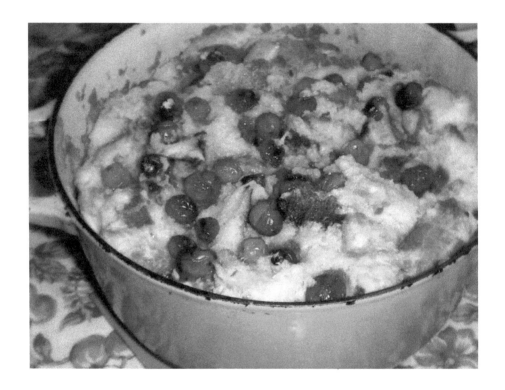

Pumpkin Chaffles

Preparation Time: 5 minutes

Cooking Time: 8 minutes

Servings: 2

Ingredients:

- 1 oz. softened cream cheese
- 1 large egg
- 1 tbsp. pumpkin puree
- 1/2 tsp. pumpkin spice
- 1 tbsp. superfine almond flour
- 1/4 tsp. baking powder
- 1/2 tsp. Erythritol granular

Directions:

1. In a bowl, stir cream cheese until it reveres a whipped consistency. If the cream cheese is too hard to whisk, melt it in the microwave for a few seconds at a time (no more than 5 seconds at a time). If you Cooking the cream cheese for too long, it will overheat and splatter all over your oven.
2. In another bowl, merge together the egg and pumpkin puree until creamy. Whisk in the pumpkin spice and almond flour until well mixed. Whether you're using baking powder and sweetener, mix them together so they're equally distributed.
3. Chaffle iron should be preheated. Grease the Chaffle iron with Cooking oil spray when it's ready.

4. Half of the batter can be poured into the mini Chaffle maker. Your batter should fill in all of the gaps. Chaffle iron should be closed. Allow for 4-5 minutes of Cooking time, or until the Chaffle is dark brown and crispy on the outside. Continue for the remaining hitter. Using the Dash mini Chaffle machine, you should have enough batter to produce two chaffles.

Nutrition:

Calories: 116.26

Carbohydrates: 2.61g

Protein: 4.52g

Fat: 9.54g

Cholesterol: 121.1mg

Potassium: 131.34mg,

Keto Pumpkin Cheesecake Chaffle

Preparation Time: 2 minutes

Cooking Time: 4 minutes

Servings: 2

Ingredients:

Pumpkin Chaffle:

- 1 Egg
- 1/2 cup of Mozzarella Cheese
- 1 1/2 tbsp. Pumpkin Puree
- 1 tbsp. Almond Flour
- 1 tbsp. of your choice sweetener
- 2 tsp. Heavy Cream
- 1 tsp. softened Cream Cheese
- 1/2 tsp. Pumpkin Spice
- 1/2 tsp. Baking Powder
- 1/2 tsp. Vanilla
- 1 tsp. Choczero Maple Syrup or 1/8 tsp. Maple Extract

Filling:

- 2 tbsp. Cream Cheese
- 1 tbsp. Lakanto Powdered Sweetener
- 1/4 tsp. Vanilla Extract

Directions:

1. Heat mini Chaffle maker.
2. Mix all chaffle ingredients in a shallow mixing bowl.

3. Set half of the chaffle batter into the Chaffle irons middle. Allow for 3-5 minutes of Cooking time.

4. Remove carefully and repeat with the second chaffle. Set aside to crisp when preparing the filling.

5. Mix all frosting ingredients in a mixing bowl with a whisk or fork. Between the two chaffles, spread frosting. Have fun!

6. Optional toppings include whipped cream, crushed pecans, and Choczero maple syrup.

Nutrition:

Calories: 231

Carbohydrate: 2g

Fat: 18g

Protein: 13g

Pumpkin Spice Chaffles

Preparation Time: 2 minutes

Cooking Time: 12 minutes

Servings: 3

Ingredients:

- 1 cup of mozzarella cheese
- 2 tbsp. almond flour
- 1 tsp. baking powder
- 2 eggs
- 1/2 tsp. pumpkin pie spice
- 2 tsp. of Swerve

Directions:

1. Mix the eggs, almond flour, mozzarella cheese, baking powder, pumpkin pie spice, and swerve in a shallow mixing bowl.
2. Pour the mixture into a small food processor and heat until smooth.
3. Cooking for 3-4 minutes with 1/3 of the batter in your mini Chaffle maker. Cooking the remaining batter to produce a second chaffle, and then repeat until all of the pumpkin spice chaffles have been made.
4. Serve with a drizzle of swerve confectioners sweetener or low carb syrup and butter.

Nutrition:

Calories 90

Fats 3.32g

Carbs 2.97g

Net carbs 2.17g

Protein 12.09g

CPSIA information can be obtained
at www.ICGtesting.com
Printed in the USA
BVHW091045090621
609091BV00008B/816